MW00443221

RE: RE:

MIDDLE, BEGINNING, END, AND REPEAT

RE: RE:

MIDDLE, BEGINNING, END, AND REPEAT

Noah Winston

RE: RE:

www.noahwinston.com

10 9 8 7 6 5 4 3 2 1

ISBN: 978-0-578-44713-1

Library of Congress Control Number: 2019900375

Photography by Noah Winston

I DON'T KNOW ANYMORE.
I CAN'T STAND THE FEELING OF NOT FEELING.

Introduction

I have a problem with understanding people. I have more of a problem with mental health. The idea of love doesn't register with me, and I am genuinely alone in this world. I'm not all about a tradition like writing an intro to a book to woo my audience. I do plan to allow you to read the things that were once in my head.

This eight by five you're holding is my journal; this is my late night tweet and drunk message to you. I want to talk to you about living with depression and anxiety, losing someone you care about even if it was just a walk in the park, dealing with family and forgiving them, pretending and showing/seeing many faces from those who call you their friend, and many more things.

I write this book for those who are like me. I write this for those who are alone and have no one to talk too. Please use this book as a way to jumpstart the emotions that's build up inside of you. Take these words to heart because that's what this is—bits and pieces of my heart cut out just for you.

I am not a poet. I am an imaginative, narrative writer who cares not about tradition. I care less of the format, the social norm to follow. I only care to write what makes sense to me. I care to share my pain for all to see in this short, compact book.

Read this book and enjoy it, hate it, despise it, and when you finish reading do whatever the hell you want with it; place it on the bookshelf and never reread it, burn it, write your book, share it with your friends and family—"I DON'T CARE" —Thebe Kgositsile.

—The Author

Contents

Middle

Your Name Belongs Here

I think ultimately I might've been heartbroken. I try and try to fight against the dark thoughts that continue to persuade me. No matter how I feel about it, everywhere I look I'm always reminded of our time spent. It may have been short, bumpy, hesitant and joyful, but it was the best time I've had in years. I felt more attached than I've ever felt towards my family, I loved more than I should my mother, and I beg for your nurturing comfort.

It's not like me to feel those things. For I despise those characteristics—*love is false hope.* I guess it's only natural seeing I'm only human. I remember you use to say some weird stuff. I didn't know what you meant. I showed the face of someone who didn't care but secretly did. I wanted to cut open your head and steal your thoughts for my own. I knew you were still discovering yourself and I had appreciated that. For I was too.

I told myself, I told my friend, I told my heart that I found someone who was just like me. Someone lost and looking for themselves. Even if we're convinced that we already found ourselves. Before we met, I was in a toxic arena with some of the worst enemies I've come to face; alcoholism, drug abuse, several suicide attempts, homicidal thoughts, discomfort, and many other troubling things. Like I said, you being here was all I needed to keep myself sane. And just like that, you left. I can't control my feelings as well as I use to. I'm not able to correctly pretend like I don't care.

I generally feel alone in this world. I learned that no matter who comes they'll always leave, whether it's my fault or theirs. I may have stopped doing things that potentially killed me, but I can't stop what's genetically in me. Seeing pictures of you or with someone else makes my stomach turn, and I just wanna break something. I can't continue to watch you from afar, so I'm deciding to let go. Knowing that I can't! This may not affect you, seeing how you always say it's easy for you to let go and cut others off, or "it's about the experience." I just wish you the best of luck in this cruel world. Hopefully, sooner or later I find what I'm looking for as you have found what you're looking for or so you thought.

Invasive Privacy

I pretended to speak your language with someone else's face on. I wanted to know how you were doing without giving away my identity.

I tried to spread you false information to corrupt your trust. In all I wanted...I needed to see what would happen.You were confused, but you also understood that the things being said were false. I ended up hurting myself trying to hurt you.

I walked into a fire thinking I was invincible. That no matter how close I was the flames could never reach. I was wrong again, and that same night I slept quietly with the reassurance that you were okay.

When I sleep

I went to sleep and woke up to a voicemail
My head was rebooting from my last standby
It was a message from me but an intoxicated version of me
This version of me expressed his feelings for me
He told me nice things and how he cared for me
He said to me

"I wished the best for you."

This didn't sound like me, but all I hear is me
He cried several times talking of the love we
share and the common mistakes we make
and that our heartbreak is one sided
He laughed at me for wanting a better life
At the end of the voicemail, I realized it wasn't me
speaking about me
It was for some girl who name I can't speak
My tongue twisted and turned
I cried feeling weak
I died a little inside
I said to myself crying back to sleep

"I wished someone cared for me, the way drunk me cares for her."

Me and you

I have a fear of rejection, so I don't claim you.

I have a long history of depression, so I don't claim you.

I have a problem with drinking and an anger disorder, so I don't claim you.

I have a distance from here to the moon between me and my family, so I don't claim you.

I don't claim you because I don't want you to hurt me mentally and I become unstable to know what's right and what's wrong.

I refuse to be attached only to one day attack the one I care about.

I don't want to build a family with you knowing I don't even attempt to sustain the bridge between mine.

There's too much at risk, so I don't. I won't. I refuse to claim you.

OBSESSED

You can't claim to be in love with someone you've only met for a few weeks to a few months. You don't love him/her you love the idea of the said person. Ask yourself what that person would do for you and what that person will not do for you. Someone can tell you down to the micro info about themselves to you but it doesn't mean they love you nor should you keep telling yourself you love them. You may know "of" their conditions, traumatic past, weaknesses, strengths, etc. but that doesn't qualify as love.

Stop fooling yourself into believing "it'll be different this time," "h/she is nice and not like the others," "h/she actually understands me and cares." It'll always be the same episode. You just watched it so much you know what to say and what not to say. If you can't destroy something as much as you build it up did you actually even care to what conditions it was in the first place? Obsession is a disease often mistaken as love. I was never in love but somewhat obsessed. I was obsessed with the idea of her, the smell of her, the ignorance and arrogance she bestowed. You are me as I am you...human and together we're OBSESSED.

BLAME GAME

I can't blame you if this isn't the lifestyle you envisioned for yourself. You're so used to the gutter, and anything besides that would be a fairytale for a princess, and you are no princess but rather a queen who doesn't know her own worth. So you hide behind the filth you call friends and family. And you silently cry when nobody's looking, and you instead have petty intercourses to fill the endless void in your heart. You lost yourself during your first love, and you haven't been the same since then. But that's no excuse to be so deprived of yourself.

ILL TELL YOU

If I had the chance, the chance to make you realize I'll tell you that not everything is about you.

I'll tell you to please refrain yourself from thinking you matter to the point that everything that comes out of my mouth is about you.

I'll tell you that I moved away from your mess because nothing you've ever told me was the truth. It's been nothing but lies, and I don't know why I eat that shit up. No matter what I say or do you'll always be the same.

I'll tell you that you'll always live the same. Feel the same. And, unfortunately spreading the same bullshit everywhere you go.

Your actions differ from your words, and that's sad. Somethings that come out of your mouth is pretty decent, It's beautiful, something I enjoy, but it's fucked that none of it will ever amount to shit.

I know I have my moments and that someone like me got problems that can't be explained and a fucked up mental state but at least, at least I can own up to the bullshit I create. I don't just talk about things I want to do. I fucking do them. Why? Because I'm a man of my word even if it's like yours and means little. Don't bother sending me any of your pictures of bullshit readings or your fake ass five syllable response.

Because I'll tell you none of that matters and you'll tell me it does and I'll tell you it doesn't, and we'll go our separate ways.

Keep Me Sane

Imagine one day you meet someone via-e then a few days later you make contact. Your boyish habits are brought to the table. The next day you become a man and let your hormones take over. A few days pass and you think to yourself,

"I don't want this to be the only thing I'm known for,"

So you try and make plans. Plans go to hell, but hey she still came over. She's un-interested In what you have to offer. So you suggest her a solution. This solution is constantly repeated meet after meet. Your tired and you just want to talk.

Your previous addictions are creeping and making weird noises in your head. You become emotional and then attached. She leaves and doesn't call. You wonder and wonder where she could have gone. Still no answer. You finally hear back from her only It's too late. Someone else is there. Your frustration is increasing. Your addiction is at an all-time high.

You nearly kill someone just because they spoke to you wrong. Then one day you drink yourself to sleep. Wake up the next morning and numb your pain with pills. Life is good. Except you're running out of pills. Those pills were the only thing keeping you sane. Now they're all gone.

Cupid

I thought that you were gone for good.
Just when the pain you gave me settled down in the pit of my
stomach.
You show up at my door,
With that smile that killed me a thousand times over,
as if nothing happened
I pretend like I don't care, but deep down inside I do.
I tried to put on a facade, one that not even I could fall for,
so instead,
I broke down
I told you how you broke me.
How you violated me.
Not in a sexual nature but much worse.
Mentally you raped me and left my mind naked.
Unclothed, limp, and bloody.
My trust, hospitality, my will to take another breath,
all taken from me because you were too selfish to realize
that your actions were hurting.
I was vulnerable
I felt like I was left on display for the world. I felt dehumanized.
By you.

4;

Strike one: Death-by-cop

During high school when I was feeling lonely and depressed, I had no one other than myself to speak to. I felt trapped within my own mind, and I had nowhere else to go. Then one night I panicked, and without reason, my mother called for help. Two cops approached me standing in my bedroom.

I decided this was it, this is where I'll do it. I reached under the bed grabbing a brass knuckle. The plan was simple you see, there were two cops. One was a heavy set male, and the other was a short feeble woman. I figured if I went for him and then she would have to come after me, so I did.

I was a lot stronger and more prominent in comparison to her so her best result would be a gunshot wound. Before lapping into action, I took one long look at my mother. I had convinced myself of moving forward but I couldn't. My legs wouldn't move an inch.

Strike two: Goner X Jack X Supply

I tried to overdose on pills and alcohol. Again I was feeling depressed and unwilling to live. I was sitting on a friends coach watching TV. Next thing I knew both hands were filled. One with a fifth of Jack and the other with an ounce of pills. I devoured what I thought to be my last supper. It didn't work, and I felt stupid. I just laid there and wondered what's next.

Strike three: Dull Knife

~~Wrist cutting isn't as easy as I thought it to be.~~

Strike four: Should've been you

I was feeling down and that none of my accomplishments in life actually mattered. That no matter who I meet or who I'm with they seem to always leave and in the end, I'm pretty much alone. I had drunk five bottles and took some pills. Put two holes in my apartment wall and tried to hang myself.

My mother called the police on me, and it was about 6-9 police cars looking for me. They locked me up in a psyche-ward. That's probably the safest I've ever felt that night, knowing I was living in reality and not another dream.

Beginning

Pawn

I was once a prince who was kidnapped by enemy warriors. I was held captive, transported from hideout to hideout. I was told what to do and when to do it. They gave me a false mother and sometimes a fake father. They made me a poster boy for the world to see.

"This is what happens when you let your guard down!" They shouted so bravely.

I had new siblings, 3-4 sisters, and 2 brothers. They kept me company until I was rescued; They too were held against their will. We were all helpless until someone came to our aid.

No Resolve

I never understood why, nor did I ever want too.

I stripped away all attachments and threw away all my perks.

I walk blindly into a world without fear, hate, or Intuition.

I am an empty shell that others pour their liquids into, to only find out I am filled with holes; therefore, I retain nothing.

I drain every last bit of what's given like the sewage beneath my feet, yet

In the end, there remains dried up residue polluting my insides like ammonia.

Echo in the Dark

Growing up I was afraid.

I was afraid to open my door at night and see the red glowing eyes in the shadows with a cricketing sound lounged in the echo.

The walls vibrated, and the air was heavy with a disease. Everything felt moist and swampy like an old Southern creek.

I close my door, but it's too late. It reopens with the presence of unwanted fumes. The voice in the shadow ask me:

"⬜⬜⬜⬜⬜⬜?," I replied with, "Yes."

Then the door closes and the weight of the air shifts and becomes breathable.

Not Yet Rated

Life is like a movie whereas everything is scripted,
and we must read word for word—
Sometimes I forget my lines because I'm too
distracted by my audience.
I can't wait to get back to my trailer and powder my face.
I hide the dark lines and red blemishes.
I don't have hair and makeup because they might notice my
insecurities. They might secretly be working for a publisher,
waiting for me to slip and tell the world of me;
All my dark secrets and sad moments exposed.

Forsaken Mother

When I was younger, I would never give my mother my school slips for parent-teacher conferences. It wasn't that I had terrible grades or misbehaved. I was sort of just afraid and embarrassed.

My mother grew up in a neighborhood most didn't or wouldn't even bother walking near at night and rarely in the day. My mother raised on discipline and a structure that made her who she was. In terms most would call her "GHETTO" and I hated that word.

It was like categorizing her in her genre of people, and it felt weird. I was shy and embarrassed to show her around. I would be terrified if she opened her mouth around others because like the current me she has no filter.

As I got older, I had become angry at myself. I had tried so hard to push my mother to be something that she wasn't, and I hadn't realized that I was making her out to be the enemy. I should have realized that it was okay for her to be her.

It wasn't nor should it be embarrassing to be who you are. I wish that I had uplifted my mother on being her rather than try to bring her down for what I considered to be her con rather than her pro.

O My Brother

Brother o brother
Brother o brother
You're so brave and kept me safe.

Brother o brother
Brother o brother
You stayed by our side even though we weren't safe.

Brother o brother
Brother o brother
If I haven't said it yet, I'll say it now. You're the best, bravest
brother of them all. You make me smile.

Brother o brother
Brother o brother
Why aren't you moving? What's wrong?

Brother o brother
Brother o brother
I hope you're well and staying strong.

Brother o brother
Brother o brother
I'm proud to call you my brother for you're strong,
and the bravest of them all.

TALES OF TALES

Amongst many, you were the very first I decided to drink from. I drank from your wishing well, wishing you well and hoping you never stopped providing for if you ever dried up, I'll die of de·hy·dra·tion.

You were like the origin of youth giving me life making me feel younger and younger with every sip I took. Then one day I drank too fast, and there were no more left. None, zip, notta.

You were dried up, and I was left wanting more. Crying as my ribcage squeezed against my bagpipes sqxueezing out dust begging for life. When I arise, someone else was tossing coins into your hole—making THIER wishes from your wishing well. I wish you well.

Wilting

Occasionally I cry at the
the idea of growing old and
perishing,
It's like for a
split second I become mortal
and think like a HU-MAN.

I

I forgive you for all the wrong you've done.
I forgive you for breaking your neck for me.
I forgive the times our plates were empty, and so were our stomachs.
I forgive you for the cold nights in the winter and the hot nights in the summer.
I forgive you for going away for 3-6 months and returning.
I forgive you for the beating you called discipline.
I forgive you for getting us back while imprisoned In a system filled with misfits.
I forgive you and your habits.
I forgive you because I hold no grudge towards you.

I hold no anger in me to spread.
I have no room to keep reminiscing about the past.
I have no time to cry over such memories, for those memories help me continue. It makes me a stronger me and how to improve what's left of me.
I have grown in so many ways because of you, so I forgive you.

Why I decide to drink

To sleep, I drink
To feel, I drink
To cry, I drink
To go on loving every single day of my life,
I must drink for if I don't—Well, I die.

After Effect

The most interesting conversation
we had didn't take place until
I reached the bottom of the bottle.

End

Farewell

There's a lump in my throat, A ball of air preventing me from swallowing, because I'm wallowing in a sea of my own emotions and there's no shoreline within miles.

Could this be my last night and if so know that I care about you, and I wish you were happy, and never have to deal with the anxiety of wanting to be free as you are as free as me when I take my last breath,

moreover, no longer singing alone in a cage like a bird with its wings cut off, or home alone, but just judging by the tone you have someone to keep you warm in this frigid world.

Wide Awake

Sometimes a little trauma helps
With sleep deprivation,

Sometimes a little clarification helps
With understanding what they call "meaning,"

Sometimes a little "hey" helps
With the idea that you care,

Sometimes a little hug helps
With the notion that you enjoy my touch.

I am kind

I hate the existence of humankind,
for humankind is not kind.
Humankind destroys,
Humankind betrays,
Humankind sells hopes and dreams of a kinder
world created by men,
but Humankind
can't create when it destroys.
Humankind is GOD.

Dear Brandy

I have always loved you, and cared more about you than life itself.
We've been together since I was like sixteen,
I remember the first time you took the air out my mouth,
The first time you gave me a taste,
it was like acid bubbling on the tip of my tongue
I've kept you by my side, through all my highs and lows in life.
You gave me the emotional comfort
and the support others couldn't give,
Mainly because you knew what I needed,
Mainly because deep down you caused it,
Damn, I'm addicted to the curves and smell that caress itself around
the spiral tip of your neck,
That sometimes is laced with thin layers of gold,
sometimes red wax dripping down your spine,
Moreover, sometimes in different flavors,

ah yes,

That flavor, what is that flavor?

Mind Your Thoughts

I got tired of displaying this weird version of me. I felt lazy, and I wasn't doing what I was supposed to do.

Sometimes you have to get rid of things that only worsen your entire being like drugs, alcohol, partying, and negative energy from people.

I went to a bookstore and read some art books, I started writing more poetry to better express myself, and went M.I.A. I isolated myself from the world to manage myself better.

I did this without friends or family...no one. I strengthened my mind and controlled my thoughts the best way I could.

A Meeting With Death

One morning I felt a ray of light on the lid of my eyes. I felt the warmth of death touching my neck, kissing me softly. I chuckled as Death tells me.

"I've found a place you can call your own."

I replied, "Is it big enough, have I heard of this place, where is it located?"

She replied gently while griping my neck,

"It's big enough, big enough for the world. You've heard of it many times indeed, You won't miss it, for it can't be missed, only those who go there."

I chuckled once more with relief, wanting to visit
She revealed,

"You'll cry an infinity before a single teardrop leaves one's eye, a cry of joy that is, because you'll finally have that rest, but only by my side."

So then Death said her goodbyes.

Feelings Not Mutual

I dreamed the impossible. Something that can never be,
I dreamed of us like two sewing threads entwined into the leather that
was once the skin of a python
I dreamed a forced smile that I couldn't acquire on my own
My charm and voice alone wouldn't even crack a smile so,
why would it in my dreams?
What makes me special?
What is it about me I ask! What is it that I can offer to her, to you?
How can I make you understand how I feel?
How I want a touch from the person, I want the most.
My lust is a secret to be kept,
secret for if it were made public, I would be the poster boy of
comedy.
I would be the joke that was never funny.
I would be the irritable caught in the corner of thy eye—
My presence only needed to being appreciated for your journey,
accomplishments you've gained and nothing else.
Sometimes I dream what if I just left this world.
Would I be missed?
Would people finally see me and my accomplishments?
Would you finally realize,
that the only way to make you hear me, see me, and feel me as I do things
that hurt us both?
I don't know anymore. I can't stand the feeling of not feeling.
I want to be comforted in ways that only you know how to. This isn't a
confession. It's a way to secretly share that I am a coward scared to go
after what I can't have. Thank you for listening.

Memory Book

Tucked away in my chamber of secrets lies a book,
This book contains memories of my greatest adventures,
This book contains memories of my toughest challenges,
This book contains memories of my happiest moments,
This book contains memories of my saddest times,

So why are you of all people in it?
Ah yes,

This book now contains my first ever love,
This book now contains my first ever heartbreak,
This book now contains my first ever sexual discovery,
This book now contains my first ever obsession,

However, what makes you unique? What requirements did you meet?
Ah yes,

You were the first to make me feel special,
You were the first to make me wanna live,
You were the first to make me lose my mind,
You were the first to make me emotionally happy,

However, this book is for the most significant moments,
Ah yes,

Like the time I marched down the streets with half a million
women in DC,
Like the time I went to prom and danced for the first time,
Like the time I cried watching Les Misérables live,
Like the time I first watched Bennington perform,

So what does this mean for me? I finally acknowledging the— "time spent?"

Is it sexual? Was it just the "experience?"

Like the time I touched your insides with two fingers, while
rubbing your clitoris,

While I drank from your breast in search of vitamins, protein, and fat,
Moreover, moving my index finger in and out of your mouth playing with
the inner wall of your gums?

Is this why? It must be more than that! Maybe it's the portrait you painted
of me, voraciously sucking the labia closes to yo-you...I think we get the
picture.

Ah yes,
It's because I'm finally able to put away another memory into the...no,

Into my "Memory Book."

In the End

In the end, you might feel alone

However, always remember that I'll still comfort you at night and tell you stories and we can laugh as we used to and star gaze into each other's eyes and dream the impossible.

In the end, you might feel unwanted

Just remember that you aren't alone, that someone is waiting for you at home and that you have someone who loves you for who you are no matter your shape, your size, or how bad your breath smells in the morning.

In the end, you might feel discomfort

I have the room set to 60° with the biggest, warmest comforters you can imagine with a bowl of your favorite ice cream lying beside you while I curl my fingers through your hair and tell you how your presence soothes me.

In the end, you might feel tired and stressed

Just know I understand how hard you work and that every time you leave, it's to further your career and make yours and my life more straightforward because we need it for what's to come when she arrives.

RE: RE:

This is the end of the road, And I thank you all for making it through my fucked, miserable, and hopeless attempt to make you feel for me. I hope you enjoy the cringe-worthy torture of hearing (reading) how incapable I am of love and how I cry at the slightest notion of someone not liking me. I thank you for staying. I thank you because you've made witness at my attempt to become famous. This is the first time pouring my heart out in papers—digitally.

"Ah yes" is what I say before I ramble on, and on about how memory serves me right. This isn't even the ending; it's the outro to an intro of more ~~fucked up~~ confusing things in my life that can one-day amount to dog level shit that nobody wants to pick up in bookstores. Also, being forced to eat greens that you've never heard of and recently found out that it might kill you because a lousy mix of chemicals sprayed on it comparable to my grief, stress, and recollections of others and how I seem to make every good thing turn virulent.

I'm not a poet—I'm an imaginative, narrative writer with a reasonable amount of trauma from adolescence memories to to high school memories and institute memories, and memories that I refuse to bring to account because it'll make me seem more stupid and trying to attempt...wait, I stuttered just a moment ago. How is it even possible to stutter—Digitally? Let me explain to you what this is while I still have the chance. I feel the alcohol running through my veins and making way to the depository of memories that serve me right, ah yes. At the end of 2017, I found out I had a twin, yes a twin! She grew up nearly the same as I did.

She too was brought up in the care of a foster mom and dad, and she too was forced to move and move to home and home with new people she's never met before. Only to one day be reunited with her I mean the drug and alcoholic infested household that birthed 6 strong negro children raised off of cornbread and skinned the bones of chicken shit called KFC short for who knows what. Ah yes, but....

Not to skip ahead but I just wanted to tell you about another girl I later met at the end of December in 2017. She taught me how to properly please a woman and hold her tight like she was being dragged away from six goblins. Sorry if that doesn't make sense now but surely it will later—but yeah, she taught me the things I always avoided in life. E.g., Love, Happiness, Attachment, and many more. I feel in love...yeah LOVE with another HU-MAN. Who would've thought? However, yeah, she made me feel happy and made me want more from life, and moments later she took those feelings away from me. It triggered something deep in me that I, nor my family have seen in years...5 years to be exact. I went on a binge drinking contest with me and my buddies; me, myself, and I.

we drank 4-6 wine bottles mixed with 2-3 bottles of vodka and went into a childish rage that had me tying six foot in length to be EXACT of rope around the bars of my apartment stairwell three floors above ground.

I played 'do or don't' with my life for about two and half hours deciding if I should hang myself and save everyone the trouble of my existents or sit there on the phone with my mum and cry and lie about everything being all right. It was all a farce because about 9 police officers surrounded me and tried to calm me before I tried anything. I gave up and allowed them to take me back home—The psychiatric hospital that is.

Things eventually have gotten better you know. I don't mean to skip timelines randomly, but things eventually have gotten better. I graduated with my associate's degree and a bachelor of fine arts degree. Things eventually have gotten better. I spent about 30/60K on a college degree that eventually took me nowhere, but I'm still here praying—*I don't pray, I'm atheist*—that things eventually get better.

My depression is getting worse, and I have nowhere to go. I refused to take my meds is the excuse I give everyone but the truth is my doctor up and left without giving me any notice, and I've been off them for about two plus years now. I left my apartment and roomed up with a friend but I long to go back home to sweet O Bay Area and still live a miserable life surrounded by those who supposedly care for me. My feelings for one of my friends have grown. I secretly creep her out, and she's not strong enough to tell me that she knows. I dream of her every other night, but let's not get off topic because eventually, things get better if I stay on track right? I do hope all of you enjoyed my rant. Like I said before I'm not a poet, I'm an imaginative, narrative writer with "a reasonable amount of trauma from adolescence memories to to high school memories and institute memories" Damn, did I copy and paste? That's lazy and unethical for a writer. Who cares these days though?

Sincerely,

Noah King "Lathan" Solomon Winston

Things eventually got worse.

Repeat

The 'ifs' and 'maybes.'

One day I won't be
obsessed with you anymore but,
until that day comes I'll
always think about the
"Ifs and maybes"
that we could've had.

Craftsman

At the time I had
refused to bring you into
My life, I refused to
use my talents and skills
to spend countless hours, blood, sweat, and
guidance from my
peers to craft such beautiful
work with you as my subject.
Knowing you would leave,
having nothing but camera roll images,
a bracelet that still smells like you,
and explicit memories had already driven me mad,
insane to the point of ending
myself staring at a photo
of you made with the
hands of Davinci and portrayed
as if Poe directed the set.

I AM WHAT I AM BECAUSE OF WHAT I AM NOT

Every bit of life if I might say is difficult
We, I, They, He, She, Meets new people who are only temporary

She plays with the hearts of men because men play with the
hearts of women

He is disloyal because he is afraid to be bound and put to the test of
honor

They pronouns changed on their 17th, 18th, 19th birthday but remain
gender-biased

I remain depressed, heartbroken, uncomfortable with
"REALITY" and tortured by cardinal sins

We lie, we destroy, we betray, we hate, we...we are hu-man
nothing more, nothing less but hu-man!

I AM NOT BECAUSE OF WHAT I AM

I LONG FOR THE TIMES SPENT, AND I CRY BECAUSE YOU
DECIDED TO END IT ALL
I DESIRED EVERY BIT OF YOUR SCENT, YOUR TASTE, AND
YOUR SMILE
I WANTED YOU TO MYSELF AND WOULD END US IF NEED BE
FOR I COULDN'T WATCH AS AN OFF BRAND VERSION OF
ME SWOOP YOU OFF YOUR FEET
I WOULD'VE GAVE UP EVERYTHING JUST TO BE BY YOUR
SIDE
I HAD NO INTEREST IN GODLY THINGS, MATERIAL
THINGS, AND PHYSICAL THINGS OTHER THAN YOU
AFTER YOU LEFT, I WAS FILLED WITH ANGER AND
WANTED EVERYTHING TO BURN
I COULDN'T UNDERSTAND ANYTHING OTHER THAN
DESTRUCTION
I WAS EVEN MORE ANGERED BY THE COMPANION YOU
KEPT BY YOUR SIDE
HE WAS A FARCE, A CHURL COMPARED TO ME
I RESENT EVERYTHING ABOUT YOU EVEN IF IT'S JUST I
LOOKING IN THE MIRROR

límbico

Deep down inside my temporal
lobe lies an "affectionate list,"
of names I made a promise
not to pursue. today one
of them escaped and persuaded
me to chase after so
I followed, following into a
a trap of my own making
I awoke naked, lying side-by-side
this repressed memory, covered in
an ounce of my own
disgust—splattered like thick chunks
of paint feeling as if
I've deflowered a sacred memory
of me and the past.
I've violated myself in order
to feel once more—
strengthening the connection between us.
stronger but It's different than before,
secretly platonic,
emotionally sexual.
I've lost sight of a
a friend and as a result
I've acquired another one.

Sometimes I Cry

Sometimes I force myself to cry because I'm not too familiar with sympathy for others.

I cry because I realize the things in life I can't obtain because of my arrogance or behavior towards others.

Sometimes I cry because I wanna throw away our friendship and spend the rest of our lives together.

Sometimes I cry because I can't understand why others mistreat you the way they do.

Sometimes I cry knowing you'll never see me the way I see you.

Sometimes I cry because I wake up with wet dreams of you
knowing they'll only be dreams.

Sometimes I cry because I know from others that your past life prevents you from experiencing the best things in life.

Sometimes I cry because you remind me of a younger version of my mother. Someone I care deeply for knowing her life as a child wasn't the best.

I cry only when I drink because my body refuses to when I'm sober, and it tells me to laugh because it doesn't know what else to do.

I cry in my sleep because I've let my guard down and my emotions run freely. I only hope I can stop crying until the day we are together.

Last Call

For the last time, you've ignored me.
Without realizing the hurt in me,
you continue to walk around freely.
I just hope one day you feel as I feel,
and recognize the chances missed
between the two of us.

Shakespeare Lullaby

I play the same scenario in my mind,
at least twice a day, I tell you,
how I feel, you looked surprised but secretly
Knew. You asked the same question every single
time, "Why are you now telling me this?"
I always reply, "The moment always slipped away."
Sometimes you laugh and tell me to shut
up, and so I do, And sometimes you
shrugged away with a grimmest look—The feeling
wasn't mutual. I arise and this time the
scenario changes, My heart is pounding away, crushed
by thy, A smile that makes me standby
and cry. So many scenarios, in time one
shall arise, Hidden in the dark it is—
Our time, our story, our beginning, our end.

DR. DR.

I don't know if it's an obsession, lust, or am I indeed In love with you. I dislike you at the same time because in my opinion you've been a neglectful friend at times and you change too quickly. I just as any man want to hug you In private and cry in your arms and pretend you're my therapist and bring you into a world of torture, so you to can understand how I feel.

Dreaming the impossible

I dreamt vividly for the first time in weeks putting aside our
friendship and explored the multiverse of what 'ifs.'

I adored the memories we shared and nearly went into car·di·ac ar·rest
just thinking the idea of your lips touching mine.

I went a little further pretending we shared the same body. My hand
was your hand touching various parts of our single body possession.

It felt like my first time all over again touching parts, discovering new
territory, kissing unfamiliar places, sliding into wet spots, superglued
to your torso as a flame burned between us.

What I tell you

I tell myself over and over that you'll be okay and you just need to hold on a little longer—someone will come to your rescue.

I keep telling myself that one day you'll be happy and the right person would come along, and all your problems will cease to exist—One day he or she will be there to support you and all your addictions.

I keep telling myself that patience is vital and that those who wait always get ahead in life—Your number has yet to be called.

But then I stopped telling you those things because I saw that you weren't okay, your happiness was still depleting, and you've waited far too long and keep having to send yourself in for repairs and that your warranty is expiring and yet you're due for another check-up.

What I tell myself

I wanna tell you the truth, and that is:

I'm here for you as a friend and would do anything to keep you safe.

I wanna be the one to make you happy and take care of you the way you should've been taken care of.

I wanna make sure every day you smile because you know you're special and that your friends and family will always have your back.

I wanna be the reason you smile and feel loved. I wanna sit by your side with friends and family and make it aware that we're meant to be.

I wanna help guide you through every heartbreak and headache from misleading people who just want to take what you have rather than give you what you need.

Hold onto that gift I gave you and when you do, always remember I'm willing and will still give to you rather than take, for when I'm with you, I have all I need.

GROWTH

Phase 1: Seeding
The first phase of your relationship was seeding. You spent countless days, weeks, and months learning each other's secrets, dos and don'ts and the things that make one another happy. Months go by, and the seed you planted into each other has split. The roots of your relationship shoot out and push down deeper into oneself. You've acquired new friends and families alike.

Phase 2: Shoot
It's been roughly a year now, and you've grown, matured enough to start thinking for two. Shortly you've been given a wider sight, your roots are stronger than ever, and you've acquired new fond memories.

Phase 3: Bud
As your relationship continues to grow, eventually, you'll start to have problems. You notice things that you didn't see at first. The truth of all your questions will slowly unfold as the sun will slowly reveal what's in the dark.

Phase 4: Bloom
In the height of your relationship, the bond that was once strengthened by the excitement, joy, and penetrating happiness seeded deep into your roots has finally blossomed into its prime. That is your happiness. Your salvation. Your knowledge for yours to keep and share with those closest to you.

Phase 5: Wilt
After a long season of beauty and life, your trust, your bond, your roots, eventually, everything will start to wilt. You'll find yourself shriveled like an infant without a mother to tend to his or her needs. All that you hold dear to you will scatter like dust in the wind into the eyes for all to see.

Phase 6: Regrowth
Once you've been stripped away from your roots and your seeds have been re-soled, you'll continue the cycle of growth once more. This time you'll grow stronger. Your roots will dig deeper than before. And you'll blossom brighter, bigger, and more beautiful than your last self. This is your resolve.

Middle, Beginning, End, And Repeat!

Day after day my mind keeps twisting with frustration. I have the same vision at least 2-3 times a week now. It's very vague and unclear, but I always see myself being hit in the mouth with an ax. Maybe it's a metaphor for something that's about to happen. The last vision involved a meat hook slicing downward from my biceps to my wrist. There's an unbelievable amount of blood everywhere, and yet I managed to live. I don't know what it is or how long it's going to last. I've been off my medication which gave me what seemed to be a voidless eternity trapped within a minute.

If anyone ever bothered to ask if I take prescriptions, I would reply, "Yes, I take antidepressants twice a day." If they pressed to ask why I tell them "I can't control my anger anymore, I feel suicidal almost every month, I have sudden urges to cry and sometimes I do. I'm used to being alone." By this time I already feel pressured. It makes me think about "family." But to be clear and bringing up the subject, since I was younger the need for a family felt pointless. They were always there, but I wasn't. I understood their roles as a mother, father, brother, etc. I just didn't feel it. Most people say it's normal. That what you're feeling will eventually disappear, but it hasn't. They said that about my depression yet it's still here.

Before my dreadful week ended, two things happened. One, I saw someone who reminded me of a carefree world. Head was filled to the brim with grace, the skin was softer than ash, and face was more memorable than the dead. As for the other, I gathered around a group of amazons and watched them breathe fire. They roared as loud as they can and continued to do so for hours. I saw a playground with sheep. Some black, some white. And some in between. They too were loud. Not in high numbers but in spirit. And finally, I was lectured by a 1000 faceless fathers and sisters. I was worried for a bit. I nearly lose my face as well. But I kept things together. I have lots and lots of new memories. I only regret sharing them alone.

This has been the longest time I've gone without writing. Between being caught in school, work, friends, and romance. I must say that this isn't the best time for me. I've gone through countless trials I might ask that will decide my fate for the rest of this year. I went two and a half weeks without contact with, who I thought to be, my better half. I've realized that this whole time it wasn't her who was wrong, but instead it was me. I fought so many years to avoid human contact. Not physically but mentally I wanted no part of emotions that would make me feel some kind of way. I learned more from that flower that blossomed one night ago than I've ever discovered, and that only a particular type of person can smell and tolerate the scent. The more I smelled, the more It reeked. It was as if I was able to see the previous people who had taken a sniff. There's so much more to talk about, but I'll leave that for another day.

Meeting With My Therapist

Growing up I never got the chance to see a doctor about my mental health; It wasn't until high school when I had my first anxiety attack. Not long after I got sent to a psychiatric ward for several weeks which eventually turned into months—I would not say I liked it. It was the worst experience at the time. I would sit up in my room at the hospital starring at the walls, and when I got home, I talked to myself for hours. I do it to this day as a coping mechanism. I find it hard sometimes to speak to others about my mental health, so instead, I created a four-part story of me talking to my imaginative therapist. I considered it to be very unrealistic, but it helped me find peace with myself at times.

Meeting With My Therapist I

DE: "So tell me...what do you fear, Either for you or another?"

DA: "...it's kind of weird you know? I don't fear much. I didn't fear anything growing up either, but once my grandfather died that changed it all. I thought I was afraid to die, but then it manifested into something else. I wasn't afraid to die I was afraid to die alone, yet that wasn't it either. When I got older, my fear grew to the purest form I guess. One that we're all familiar with. I was afraid to be alone."

DE: "Can you elaborate a little more?"

DA: "I have friends and family, but I just never felt a connection towards them. They were just there, and I was over here...I felt there was nothing out there for me and then one day... one day I found it."

DE: "what was is it that you found?"

DA: "It was a girl."

DE: "Tell me about her. What was it about her that made you feel different?"

DA: "Well she was different. They usually are."

DE: "Who is?"

DA: "The people we meet...She was weird in the beginning and talked like one of those horoscope books. I didn't understand what it meant to her or if she knew what she was saying, but I knew she believed what she was saying. She was searching for answers herself."

DE: "She sounds mesmerizing. What made you become so obsessed or were you, to begin with?"

DA: "Obsessed! Hmm, I guess she...from what I thought she was into me, but that wasn't it. She made me feel special you know? I never felt that way before, and I wanted to feel like that all the time. I don't know what it was, but there was something about her that made me feel like living. Every time we met regardless of how I felt, it all went away. All my worries, stress, regret you know? Everything ceased to exist. She was like a hard reset for my emotions if that makes any sense?"

DE: "Sounds like you were in love. However, now that I see you, you seem pretty...emotionless and tired. Why is that?"

DA: "It happens. Even though we only knew each other for a short period, it took a huge toll on me. We met at a time when I was going through a lot, and I just threw my entire self at her. I feel like I rushed everything—*I probably did*. I needed her to take control of everything. I wanted to feel dominated and yet I didn't. Time after time I started reverting to my old self. I started becoming a mean, selfish, asshole. I once tried ignoring her, but I couldn't resist hearing her voice. She caught on to what I was doing too. She sees things that I can't see myself, but I guess it doesn't matter anymore. She was gone before she saw the rest, but I feel like she knew I was hurt. If she didn't then good for her I guess. I wouldn't want to worry her with this."

DE: "You said earlier...The last time we spoke that you wrote poetry correct? Did you ever write anything about her?"

DA: "I don't make poetry per se. Sometimes I drink a lot and pick up a pen and paper, but to answer your question, yes! I've written a few times about her."

DE: "Can we hear some of it?"

DA: "Ummm I don't really like sharing them. I have them saved on my phone. They're password protected. I can let you read one-off record only though."

DE: "Okay cool, so just for today I think we have what we need. I'm glad you shared this with me."

DA: "Actually, if you don't mind I would like to share maybe one or two with you."

DE: "Okay, let's hear it."

DA: "It's called *Cupid* kind of corny haha."

Cupid

I thought that you were gone for good.
Just when the pain you gave me settled down in the pit of my
stomach.
You show up at my door,
With that smile that killed me a thousand times over,
as if nothing happened
I pretend like I don't care, but deep down inside I do.
I tried to put on a facade, one that not even I could fall for,
so instead,
I broke down
I told you how you broke me.
How you violated me.
Not in a sexual nature but much worse.
Mentally you raped me and left my mind naked.
Unclothed, limp, and bloody.
My trust, hospitality, my will to take another breath,
all taken from me because you were too selfish to realize
that your actions were hurting.
I was vulnerable
I felt like I was left on display for the world. I felt dehumanized.
By you.

DE: "That was really... something. Did you write that yourself?"

DA: "Yes. I had a friend proofread it for me though. she has a knack for it."

Meeting With My Therapist II

DE: "...Well, I'm glad to see you again, Lathan."

DA: "...."

DE: "How are you feeling today?"

DA: "I feel a little more open to speaking today. I have a lot going on and need someone to talk to."

DE: "Well I can certainly say that is the whole purpose of this, is it not?"

DA: "Yeah, and you've been a tremendous help so far."

DE: "Thank you, Lathan. So tell me what's been going on lately?"

DA: "Lately everyone and everything around me has been feeling and looking less and less real. I keep reminiscing about things that felt the most real to me. Like the time I was left on display with a knife plunged into my chest yet there was no blood to spill, and every time I think about it I feel more like a failure each waking day. I deleted images off my phone to make room and stumbled across a collection of memories that shattered me once again like the day she left, and she never gave me a when nor where. I stare constantly looking into a pit of darkness. It felt too similar to the sunken place from the film Get Out, and I felt like the images were the tea, and I was looking and looking for someone to spill it or break the glass that held all my troubles and worries in a single place. I've lost the feeling, the idea of death creeping through my window, the homicidal thoughts are no more. All that remains is the small cortex behind my brain that triggers memories and pain, and I'm just sick of the pain that keeps me...that makes me feel like everything will always remain the same. Why of all people must I feel this way? I thought I gave up on that past life. I thought that the stages of grief, forgiveness, and amongst all things heartbreak was all behind me. However, one look at the photos I keep and I turn into a scared little kid lost in a store looking for his mother."

DE: "If you had the chance to speak to her what would you tell her? How about you use me! I want you to visualize me as her and tell me what's on your mind."

DA: "For the safety of you and I, I rather not visualize you as her."

DE: "Okay, that's understandable but tell me..express yourself, Lathan!"

DA: *If I had the chance, the chance to make you realize I'll tell you that not everything is about you.*

I'll tell you to please refrain yourself from thinking you matter to the point that everything that comes out of my mouth is about you.

I'll tell you that I moved away from your mess because nothing you've ever told me was the truth. It's been nothing but lies, and I don't know why I eat that shit up. No matter what I say or do you'll always be the same.

I'll tell you that you'll always live the same. Feel the same. And, unfortunately spreading the same bullshit everywhere you go.

Your actions differ from your words, and that's sad. Somethings that come out of your mouth is pretty decent, It's beautiful, something I enjoy, but it's fucked that none of it will ever amount to shit.

I know I have my moments and that someone like me got problems that can't be explained and a fucked up mental state but at least, at least I can own up to the bullshit I create. I don't just talk about things I want to do. I fucking do them. Why? Because I'm a man of my word even if it's like yours and means little. Don't bother sending me any of your pictures of bullshit readings or your fake ass five syllable response.

Because I'll tell you none of that matters and you'll tell me it does and I'll tell you it doesn't, and we'll go our separate ways.

Meeting With My Therapist III

DE: "Today I want to start from the beginning. I was hoping you could tell me about your childhood to the best of your knowledge. Don't leave anything out and don't be afraid to go into the details of your past. I wanna hear it from you, Noah."

N: "....well...I was born and raised in California until around 11. I moved to El Dorado, Arkansas for a short period before moving to..."

DE: "I don't mean to stop you this is good info but what I wanna know is about your childhood. Tell me about you."

N: "...I am a middle child of 6, and from the moment I was born I was already pronounced dead."

DE: "I'm sorry? You were already "pronounced dead?" Elaborate a little for me I'm perplexed."

N: "Well, I was born with a heart problem, and I've had a respiratory infection since then. It comes from my father side of the family."

DE: "So you have bad health? How does that correlate with the dead part?"

N: "On my mother side of the family there's a Black Friday deal. You get chronic depression, violent mood swings, and sometimes, just sometimes paranoia."

DE: "Hmm, I understand you've had asthma your entire life but what about the mental illness? That's new right?"

N: "No!"

DE: "Maybe this was a hard question for you. I don't feel as if I know you or know of you. It's as if you don't know the answer to the question yourself."

N: "Maybe..."

Meeting With My Therapist IV

DE: "Todays our final day talking Lathan. I think that this has been quite helpful, but I also fear that we haven't covered everything. Tell me, before this end how you will show resolve?"

DA: "I've finally realized that everything is my fault. No one can make me do or act in such matters but myself. Its come to my conclusion that my entire life is the way it is because I've failed to realize my own mistakes sooner."

DE: "Why would you think everything is your fault?"

DA: "I feel as if I had given every one or everything around me a chance I wouldn't be as I am. I feared rejection growing up, so I avoided people. I feared death, so I rarely left the house. I never took the risk. I thought the human body was frail and weak compared to other species. We're walking meat bodies with soft emotions that have proven to destroy one another for the color of one's skin, for the wealth of another, for the company one keep, and some do without thought, which is even scarier."

DE: "So if you were more like everyone else you'd be a better you?"

DA: "Yes! I feel as if there's a small percentage of people like me who feel like they're the anomaly of the world. We stand out, and people noticed us. We're depressed because we're alone, separate by those a lot like us. We're sad because everyone we befriend always seem to betray us. It's as if we aren't meant to be with anyone who isn't like us."

DE: "Is that how you feel about the other girl? Do you believe that you two were never meant to be?"

DA: "Not everything in this world makes sense. Imagine two twin brothers separated at birth. Two anomalies by some miracle meet 20 years later and then two years after being reunited one of the anomalies stabs the other in the back...literally. Why is that?"

DE: "I don't quite understand. Why would one of the brothers kill the other?"

DA: "I never said kill but here's what I think. Two people exactly alike separated by birth. As I said before, "we're alone, separate by those a lot like us" but what happens when one of us are affected by those who aren't like us? What do we become? We're no longer anomalies. We're just as they're...no. We're much more now. We can no longer coexist with those like us because they have been affected by those opposite of us."

DE: "Where is this going? Where is this leading? It sounds more like a conspiracy if anything"

DA: "She was once like me but was affected by those opposite of us. She's more than what she expected to be in life."

DE: "Is that a good thing?"

DA: "...I don't know, and I'm not the one who changed she is."

DE: "How can you know she's the one who changed? How confident are you that she's the anomaly? What makes you believe you aren't the one who changes? Why Noah, Huh? Why?"

DA: "I DON'T KNOW. STOP, STOP, STOP, STOP."

Untitled A Side

When I first set out to write this book I had dozens of rough ideas I've written. I was writing down anything that came to mind that I felt could have potential. These stories or verses soon later became the reference log to writing this book. They may seem familiar because I've used some of them in a line or two throughout the book.

1. I panicked when you showed me the universe. My virgin eyes went blind.

2. I'm afraid that if I take off this mask your wearing, there would just be another one.

3. I found rest inside a black hole. My existence was no more.

4. Love is a metaphor for a child who constantly needs to drink from the torso of their mother!

5. I'm only interested in your passionate side, which I never get to see.

6. Apparently, death would be the only common interest we share.

7. Your words reached me, but deep down I knew they weren't yours, to begin with.

8. You've drained me of all my compassion. It is why I must die.

9. I damaged myself just to repair you.

10. Our reunion was a mistake, accident, according to you. But the more separated we became, the more you yearned. The more I yearned.

11. Your blossom was bitter like a rose, but the scent was that of a tulip.

12. I drank from your wishing well, wishing you well.

13. You've ignited the coal in my heart and then put me out. I'm back to my old self.

14. You've peaked my interest. Now that I am, you've gone and made me obsessed.

15. My mind is filled with memories of course, but what I like most are the bad ones. Its crazy huh? but I think the good memories can only last so long. The bad ones are usually more enjoyable. Crazy I guess. Doesn't make any sense.

16. I found something special and just like that it's gone.

17. I'm hurting far worse than I attended—please HELP!

18. I listen to your music when you aren't around. It makes me feel closer to you.

19. I thought you made yourself clear plenty of times. I just refused to listen. I was scared to face the obvious. That was—that there would never be "us."

20. In my short two decades I've only cried for four things—happiness, sadness, truth, and lies. In the end it was because of you.

21. I loaned you my heart and you returned it broken.

Untitled B Side

Just before wrapping up my last short stories I started having conflicts mentally, with friends, family, and partners. My anxiety started triggering off and on, and I had no one to speak too, no one who would listen, no one ever asked. I felt I had lost someone close to me. I eventually wanted to keep writing to keep my myself occupied, so I started writing an untitled collection of poems and short stories. I spent weeks off and on without writing and feeling as if I wouldn't finish this, but as time went on and as I drank more the memories started flowing out.

Untitled I

i try so very hard to forget you but i can't
i still hold a grudge against you for
all the love i had in me because of you
no longer exists
you and i could've been more
this isn't how i envisioned our ending
i wish we could start over.

Untitled II

i was a young man when we first met. you were experienced in things i can only wish, and then one morning i begged you for a "feel." you left, and when you came back, you showed me the universe. i panicked because my virgin eyes had seen too much. it was as if i had been eve and you were adam for i had eaten the forbidden fruit which caused us sorrow.

Untitled III

i support you in every aspect of you being you.
i want to dehumanize your entire being for just your existence.

i respectfully acknowledge who you are.
i honestly want to test my luck and pretend you aren't even real.

i don't tend to violate or strike fear in you.
i tend to do terrible things to you because i am superior to you in every aspect and want you to know you're nothing without my voice.

Untitled IV

i remember my first time. i remember the thoughts going through my head at the time and the way my heart beat increased.

i remember the room temperature and the smell of the carpet that she laid back on. the pillows were soft and warm, and the cotton squeezed out from its sides.

i remember the color of her eyes staring me down even though the room was pitch black and not a sound in miles but hers and mine.

i remember the comfort of pushing my lower side into her warm moist empty lot filled with heavy rain.

i remember the wall squeezing in on me trapping me in a tight space that made me scream aloud. i remember my neck being squeezed because her hands were free and needed to be gripped around something for safety.

i remember the sound echoing off the walls that had woken the dogs in each room.

i remember not telling her she was my first time and that it felt terrible. i remember not telling her that i was thinking of someone else the entire time we were conjoined like twins.

i remember feeling bad because i lost my motivation and felt uncomfortable. i remember not being able to look her in her eyes because i felt ashamed and shy at the same time. i remember crying by her side and covering it up with laughter to distract her.

i remember drinking from her torso because it was convenient enough that ironically i felt like a helpless child. there's so much i wish i didn't remember.

Untitled V

i feel like if i were to ask you'll say no. you might find me being funny. you probably wouldn't take my request seriously. i am the jokester, and you're my audience. i laugh it off as i do everything else and i continue to live my life without you.

Untitled VI

i'm always searching for myself at the end of some tunnel.

i'm giving up because i no longer exists.

i never pray to god/s because men created god/s.

i am a boy helping father release some stress.

i praise women to the utmost level for they gave birth to whole continents of children.

your service is no longer needed for my offspring is finally here.

i always keep an open mind because i'm optimistic.

deep down inside i still judge you because you are different and different frightens me.

Untitled VII

sometimes i lay on my side thinking of the past. i think so hard that it becomes real. the only thing is when i awake i realize it was nothing more than a dream.

every night i awake in a puddle of my tears. it's as if i've dragged buckets of water from a lake to drown myself where i lay.

Untitled VIII

i'm an open book allowing others to check me off the shelf. my neighbors are too! my favorite book whom i've known for years reads to me every night. there's soo much to learn, and i never get bored either. it's just sometimes i want to skip a few pages because i've read ahead on my own.

i want to go deeper into the pages near the index, but i'm never allowed. instead, someone else reads them to me. and before i get to hear about it at least, seven others have read it. i only had the opportunity to listen to it when it's forced.

by that time i don't even care anymore; instead, i want to read different pages from different books. every other book is boring and not as entertaining as the previous, so every night i reread my pages trying to find the interesting parts and the most important—*page 300, chapter 21, line 96. "the curious life of..."*

Untitled IX

growing up, i was told to go to church. go to school. stay on the righteous path to glory. they told me that if i make good grades and impress my peers and seniors, i'll be on my way to the top. they tell me to do what makes me happy and to find someone special to share it with. but what they didn't tell me is that the world is messy. it's filled with crooks, thieves, and greed. they didn't tell me that no matter how much you desire something someone else will take your place for cheaper expenses. that no matter how many jobs you get and how many resumes you submit that i'll never be able to meet ends needs. they did tell me, however, to go to college and make them proud. that people with degrees make the most money. they tell me so, so much, yet they don't tell me the truth. why is that?

Untitled X

i miss the choking and bruises
we gave one another
the torment and abuse fueled
my heart with
joy
and
excitement
i couldn't resist to misbehave in public
and
let others know how into you i was
i reminisce about your pain
and
suffering sometimes that i physically
abuse myself in your honor
the awkward moments
and
serious moments were always alike.

Acknowledgement

To my friends (you know who you are), family and supporters alike who have helped me build these memories and put them to good use. You all were a great group of unlicensed therapists.

I thank you all. I thank you as well ***** for if we've never met, I wouldn't have begun to pursue this emotional side of me that allowed me to express suppressed emotions. I'm thankful to be able to share the things in my life with you all.

RE: RE:

MIDDLE, BEGINNING,

END, AND REPEAT

A book of poems and short stories

by

Noah Winston

INSTAGRAM: @LATHANDAVINCI

CPSIA information can be obtained
at www.ICGtesting.com
Printed in the USA
LVHW071923160422
716384LV00017B/362